Keeping Weight Off Forever

WORKBOOK

What's your Relationship Status?
It's complicated…

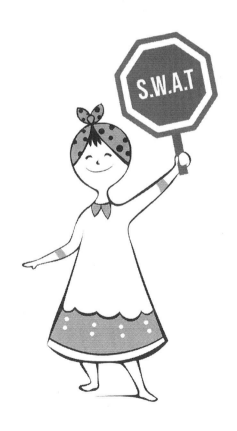

Susan Macey PhD

Printed in the United States of America

First Edition, 2018

ISBNs:
978-1-7326195-0-0 (Paperback)
978-1-7326195-1-7 (E-Book)
978-1-7326195-2-4 (Workbook)
978-1-7326195-3-1 (Journal)

Illustrations Copyright © 2018 by Stefani Truyol • stefanitruyol.com
Editing by Steven Pate
Book & Cover Design by Darlene Swanson • van-garde.com

Please address any inquiries or comments to
www.SusanMaceyPhD.com
Susan@gobeyondthediet.com
smaceyphd@gmail.com

Contents

Section Two: Aligning

Section Three: Refining

IF YOU KEEP DOING THE same things, the same things will keep happening. Changing your trajectory is one of the tenets of this workbook. What is a trajectory? It is the direction in which something will go, a path if you will. If we don't change, our trajectory will be the same. In order to have lasting change in your life, you have to understand how it is you came to do the things you do, whether it has to do with your food choices and habits or an attitude you've adopted. You didn't just arrive here in a vacuum. You got here by making choices along the way. Now, a new journey is about to begin. In this new journey, you will learn to understand your relationship to food. In order to keep your weight off forever, you have to change your relationship to food forever. To do this, you have to understand your current relationship to food. How did you get here? Now, are you willing to embark on making it a healthy relationship?

This workbook will help you think about the changes you want to make as well as give you tools to help you think about the choices and decisions you are making. Each exercise is designed to move you from where you are to where you want to be. Not all of the exercises may seem relevant to you. Just because something is difficult does not mean it should be skipped. If you choose not to do the assignments, it is likely that you won't change your trajectory. When you invest time in yourself, it will pay off in dividends.

Often people say, "Change is difficult." Yes, it can be difficult; at the same time, it is okay to be in an uncomfortable place. In order for you to make lasting changes, to make the new habits and behaviors second nature, you have to be uncomfortable. When you are working out, and your muscles get sore, guess what? You are getting stronger! Your discomfort is a sign of rebuilding, strength, and progress. In fact, when we are uncomfortable, we secrete a neurochemical that helps train the brain. Yes, that's right! Your brain has neuroplasticity, which means it can change and be rewired. However, in order for that change to take place, you have to be uncomfortable. You are the engineer of your brain. When you work towards changing your habits, beliefs, and even learn something new, your neurochemistry changes and so does the structure of your brain.

Section One: Defining

IN SECTION ONE, YOU ARE going to be practicing the art of defining. The process of defining is essential. When we define the tool, our food lane, and our behavior lane, we are creating a powerful process for commitment and ultimately change. Defining guidelines brings an awareness to ourselves and an understanding that is clear and specific. Defining is not about limitations; it's about possibilities, and opportunities. Keep in mind that how you decide to overcome roadblocks, ask questions, define your food and behaior lane is ultimately up to you.

Chapter One:
Defining the Tool

1. Identify roadblocks for change

2. Deconstruct roadblocks for change.

3. Define the S.W.A.T. method for thought stopping.

4. Practice slowing down your actions and observing.

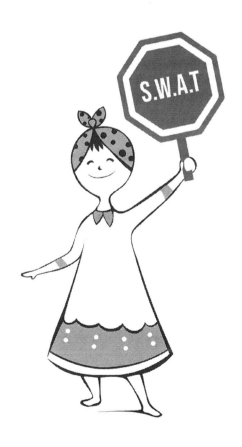

Powerful Process: Overcoming Roadblocks

Our biggest challenges in life are the roadblocks we place in our own path. Take a minute and in column one, write down the roadblocks in your path. Write down all the **reasons why you can't or won't make changes**. Most often the list is comprised of **time, money,** and **people**.

In the second column, write down how you will overcome each roadblock. Think about how you have **overcome** the roadblock in other areas of your life. Now apply that to making healthy choices.

Your perceived blocks to success	Suggestions for overcoming blocks
I have a stressful job.	I could learn to set boundaries on my time at work by eating lunch away from my desk or taking a walk outside for 10 minutes.

S.W.A.T.

What S.W.A.T. questions might you ask yourself now that you've identified your roadblocks and identified ways of overcoming them? Remember S.W.A.T. stands for: Stop What you are doing (take a breath), Ask yourself some questions, then Take action. The first step in taking action is to answer the questions and then decide on your final action. Journaling this process helps you remember your S.W.A.T. questions.

Identify the situation is column one, then write out your questions in column two. Use the third column to identify the actions you took, and how it turned out. Reflect on the process and the results of the actions in column three.

Situation I S.W.A.T.ed	Questions I asked myself	Action or Actions I took	What I might do differently next time
Example: At the church picnic tempted by cake.	Is this something that will help me achieve my goal? Would it be okay to walk away?	The action is answering the questions: Yes, it's okay to walk away, and I did.	Nothing. I did not eat the cake.

Chapter 2:
Defining Your Food Lane

1. Define the meaning of cravings.

2. Identify the underlying reasons for cravings: gut health, food sensitivity, and food addiction.

3. Create a weight loss meal plan: define your food lane.

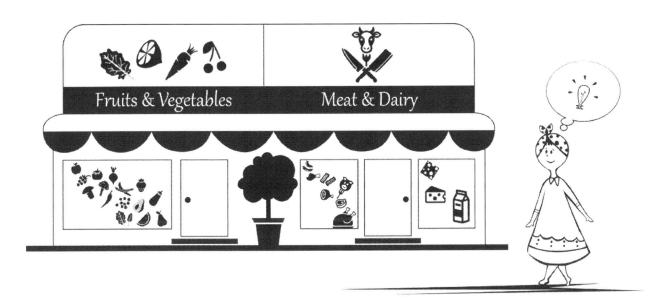

Powerful Process: Identifying the underlying reasons for your cravings

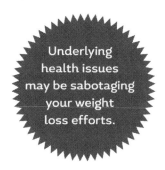

Underlying health issues may be sabotaging your weight loss efforts.

Take some time and examine how you feel after you eat. When we have been experiencing the same symptoms for so long, they are thought of as "normal." Pay attention to what types of foods you are eating and any physical response you experience.

Examine Your Gut Health			
Symptoms	Frequency		
Nausea	Never	Sometimes	More often than not
Burning in your throat or chest	Never	Sometimes	More often than not
Bloating	Never	Sometimes	More often than not
Constipation	Never	Sometimes	More often than not
Diarrhea	Never	Sometimes	More often than not
Irritable bowels	Never	Sometimes	More often than not

Many of these symptoms could indicate you have gallstones, diverticulitis, GERD, celiac disease, or irritable bowel syndrome. If you suffer from these symptoms "sometimes," keep a food journal so you can identify which foods or combination of foods are having an adverse impact on your body. Then seek medical advice.

Are there other symptoms you are experiencing? Write them down here and try and associate the types of food or foods that may have impacted that reaction.

_____

_____

_____

_____

_____

_____

Food Journal

Type of food	Time of day	How I felt after eating
Ex: Two eggs, bacon, and two slices of white bread with butter	6:00 a.m.	Felt bloated, then needed to go to the bathroom

Examine the Possibility of a Food Sensitivity

Over time we can develop food sensitivities. A sensitivity is different from an intolerance. If you have a food sensitivity, your symptoms may be non-existent one day and severe on another. Often people associate the symptoms with other things such as being tired or stressed. Our diet has a major impact on how we feel both physically and emotionally.

Examine Food Sensitivity			
Symptoms	Frequency		
Food cravings	Never	Sometimes	More often than not
Brain fog/confusion	Never	Sometimes	More often than not
Headaches/migraines	Never	Sometimes	More often than not
Depression or mood changes	Never	Sometimes	More often than not
Heartburn	Never	Sometimes	More often than not
Gas/bloating	Never	Sometimes	More often than not
Joint pain	Never	Sometimes	More often than not
Skin problems: rosacea. acne, dark circles	Never	Sometimes	More often than not

If you are experiencing the above symptoms sometimes or more often than not, then it's time to look at a possible food sensitivity. The foods at the top of the list for sensitivity are dairy, soy, and gluten. Take a look at your diet, read the labels and determine if you are suffering from a food sensitivity. Then do an elimination diet.

Foods to eliminate	Date you stopped	Observation
Ex: Dairy	3/12/18	Didn't feel bloated

Elimination diet:

A basic elimination diet consists of cutting out the food that you suspect is causing your reaction for at least eight days. Then add the food back on the ninth day. Once you do, notice if your symptoms return. Sometimes it can take eating that food for a day or two to notice any changes.

Observation when food is added back into your diet	
Example: Tomatoes	Did not feel a tingling sensation in my mouth after I ate my salad
Day 1 Experience	
Day 2 Experience	
Day 3 Experience	
Day 4 Experience	
Day 5 Experience	
Day 6 Experience	
Day 7 Experience	
Day 8 Experience	
	Add the food back and monitor your reaction. Keep monitoring your response to the food. Sometimes the response may be more about how much you are eating. For example I may be able to eat a roll, but when I eat an entire sandwich or pizza, I experience a reaction.

Examine the Possibility of Addiction to Food

Food addiction is a real thing. Most often the underlying cause is a need to be relieved from emotional pain. When you were a child, did your mother give you candy to help you calm down? When you were afraid or thought you disappointed your parents, did you reach for an extra cookie or two? Food addiction can also be genetic. If you have had people in your family who suffered from addiction, such as alcoholism, then you may be sensitive to addictive behaviors.

Identify your behaviors and thoughts regarding food, then assess the frequency.

Addiction to Food			
Behaviors/Thoughts	Frequency		
Do I resist the need to give up a certain food	Never	Sometimes	More often than not
Thinking about food or my next meal	Never	Sometimes	More often than not
Hide food or eat in secret, even in the car	Never	Sometimes	More often than not
Rationalize or make excuses for my choices	Never	Sometimes	More often than not
Feel out of control or compare my behavior to others	Never	Sometimes	More often than not
Continue the behavior despite negative consequences	Never	Sometimes	More often than not

If you suspect a food addiction, it's time to get help. Find a professional who can help you with your food addiction and the underlying reasons.

In order to begin to define your food lane, take some time and pay attention to your body's response to foods and any cravings you might experience. Use the chart below to assess how you feel after a meal. Defining our food lane for fat loss is not as simple as calories in and calories out. If a low calorie food causes you to have a negative physical reactions, this food should not be in your food lane. This journal will help you define what foods are best for you for weight loss and maintenance. In column one identify the foods you are eating, in column two, list the time of day, in column three write how you physically felt after you ate it, and finally any thoughts or ideas about the experience.

Food Journal: Journal for examining the physical effects of food.

Type of food	Time of Day	How I felt after eating	Thoughts
Ex: Two eggs, bacon, and two slices of white bread with butter	6:00 a.m.	Felt bloated, then needed to go to the bathroom	Next time eliminate the bread and butter and see how I feel

Defining your food lane

Defining your food lane for fat loss is essential to your success. Defining your food lane may take some time. Read through Chapter 2 and determine your course of action. As you complete the exercises below, you will get a good idea of what your food lane should look like. You may feel resistant to making these changes. However, for you to feel your best, these are the changes that may need to take place. Just because you are finding it difficult to make better food choices and define your lane does not mean it's time to stop practicing. This process takes time. Here is a list foods and a worksheet to help you define your lane.

Defining Your Food Lane (Fat Loss)

Daily grams of Protein _____

Daily grams of Carbohydrates _____

Daily grams of Fat_____

Section 1: Identify the protein sources that you like, how you might prepare them, and any recipe you like.

Proteins	Preparation Ideas	Favorite Recipes/ Meal ideas
Beef:	Grill	
Poultry:	Sauté	
Fish/Sea food	Crock-pot	
Lamb or Pork:	Bake	
Game:	Broil	

Vegetables	Preparation Ideas	Favorite Recipes/ Meal ideas
Broccoli Cauliflower Kale	Grill Sauté Crock-pot Bake Broil	

Dairy	Preparation Ideas	Favorite Recipes/ Meal ideas
Cottage Cheese Yogurt		

Legumes	Preparation Ideas	Favorite Recipes/ Meal ideas
Black beans Pinto beans		
Add the food items you most often eat.	Identify the many ways of preparing foods.	Make a list of your favorite recipes and keep it handy. Pay attention to flavor by adding in spices. Focus on flavors you like.

Options, Options, and more Options		
Seasonings	**Favorite Flavors**	**Dining out ideas/options**
Spices, herbs, and seasonings	Ex. Mexican	Order fajitas and skip the flour tortillas, rice, and beans
Vinegars (not balsamic)		
Mustard		Indulgences: Frequency
Stock: Chicken, beef, vegetable, mushroom, Pho		
Butter, Coconut oil, Olive oil		Other: Foods I want to include that are not on the list
Salad dressings (check the labels)		
Lemon and Lime		
Add your favorite seasonings and keep them on hand	Find alternatives to favorite foods like spaghetti and meatballs; exchange for spiralized zucchini with meat balls and crushed tomatoes	List your "go to" restaurants and find foods that are within your food lane. For example, at your favorite steak place, skip the potato and opt for extra broccoli or asparagus.

Use the list of foods you identified as your shopping list and your guidelines for when you go out to dinner. Once you begin shopping from your list, you will always have food on hand that is in your lane.

Food Log

Keeping a food log is known to increase the success rate for people who what to reduce their weight. To help determine the best dietary guidelines for you, keep track! When you want something that is not on your plan, you can use this log to help you figure out the invisible motivators behind your behavior. Keep it simple!

To determine the nutritional information, there are various applications you can download on your phone or go to www.Nutritiondata.self.com or www.AuthorityNutrition.com.

Time	Food	Carbs grams	Protein grams	Fat grams	Calories	Place	Mood	What could I have done differently?
6:30 PM	Hamburger French Fries 2 Beers	28 73.8 21.2	18 7.1 2.6	20 28.4 0	359 282 290	Local Pub with friends	Good Went along with others	Skipped the bun and fries. Have burger on lettuce. Maybe 1 beer or none

Chapter 3:
Defining Your Behavior Lane

1. Identify toxic relationships to food.

2. Establish eating boundaries and set behavior guidelines.

3. Understand hunger cues.

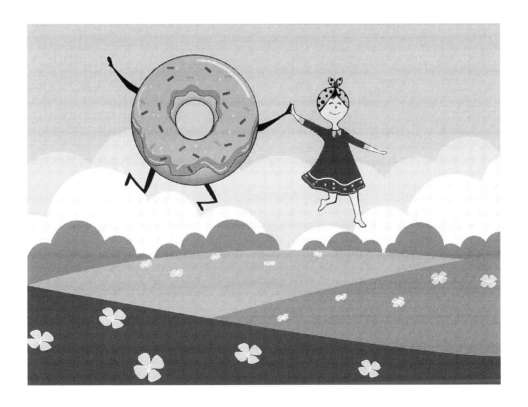

Powerful Process: The break up letter

Writing your own breakup letter is powerful. Take a few minutes and reflect on what food item or behaviors have been there for you.

What was or has been your go-to food?

What were the situations where you chose that food?

How were you feeling? How did eating it make you feel?

What was good about the relationship? What was bad?

What have you learned?

Dear _____

_____

_____

_____

_____

_____

_____

_____

Powerful Process: Settting New Guidelines

Think about your eating behaviors. Are there some guidelines you feel would be helpful to incorporate into your life? *The goal* of this exercise is to think about your old patterns and begin to establish a new guideline. Once you do that, you can practice keeping within the guideline.

Powerful Process: Setting New Guidelines

Identify a pattern of behavior you do that you know sabotages your goals.

Write down a new guideline for that behavior. Then over the course of a week, practice that guideline. If it works for you, great. If not, come up with a new guideline.

Old Pattern of Behavior	New Guidelines
Example: Eating in my car on the way home from work	No eating in the car: Drinking water in the car
Eating at my desk	Eating at the table and taking at least 10 min to finish my lunch.

Remember these are guidelines, not rules. They can be flexible when you need them to be, not necessarily when you want them to be. S.W.A.T to make sure you are making the best possible choices at any given time.

23

Understanding Hunger

It's easy to get confused between wanting and needing food. Over time we assume that much of what we are feeling is hunger. Take a day and monitor how you are feeling; every hour notice if you are hungry. Get to know your body's hunger cures. Take a minute and write down how you know you are hungry.

What do you experience when you are hungry?

Mildly Hungry: _____

_____

_____

_____

_____

Moderately Hungry: _____

_____

_____

_____

_____

Extremely Hungry: _____

_____

_____

_____

_____

_____

As you go through your day, ask yourself, "Am I hungry?" If so, is it mild, moderate, or extreme? If you are unsure, take a day and monitor yourself every hour:

Time	No Hunger	Mild-H	Mod-H	Ex-H	How am I feeling
6:00 AM	Ex: √				Relaxed and calm
7:00					
8:00					
9:00					
10:00					
11:00					
12:00 PM					
1:00					
2:00					
3:00					
4:00					
5:00					
6:00					
7:00					
8:00					
9:00					
10:00					
11:00					

Lifestyle Review

Many people believe that in order to get healthy, lose weight, and keep it off forever, they need a "lifestyle change." Wow, a lifestyle change? That seems a bit extreme to me. When I think about making a lifestyle change, I imagine a complete overhaul of my entire life. Even a 60,000-mile tune-up doesn't involve replacing your entire engine. Let's face it, changing your entire life is not going to happen, and the good news is that it doesn't have to. You don't need a complete overhaul in order to achieve your goals and maintain your weight. Take a minute and think about your life.

Exercise: Lifestyle Review

Sit comfortably and relax your body, face, and eyes. As you do, reflect on the full span of your life.

Notice how your life has changed over the years. You can conjure up images of when you were a child going to elementary school, riding the school bus. Later you were able to walk to school and then drive to school. Eventually, you see yourself owning your own car and being completely independent.

With each change came a new set of responsibilities as well as freedoms. You can see how you developed and changed, as did your lifestyle. It happened gradually.

Some of the changes were scary, to be sure, especially as you've taken the leap into adulthood: working full time, maybe married, or raising children.

What are you noticing about your lifestyle?

How do you spend your time?

Powerful Process: Life Style Review and Options

What can't change?	Problem	What do I want?	Possibilities
Example: Long Commute	One hour commute each way to work. No time to exercise	I want to be able to exercise 2 days a week.	1. 2 days a week walk at lunch 2. 2 days a week stay later after work and walk for 20 min. 3. Join a nearby gym
I Have a 2-year-old	When I get home from work, he is hungry: I need to play with him, and then it's bedtime. No time for me to eat a healthy meal.	I want to cook and enjoy a healthy meal and spend time with my child.	1. Feed the baby a snack while you prepare a healthy meal. 2. Eat dinner first as a family, then play time, then bath time. 3. Switch off between parents preparing dinner.

Chapter Four:
Defining Course Correction

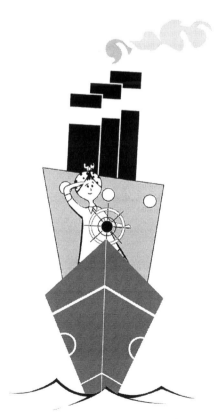

A different view gives you a new perspective on possibilities

Powerful Process: New Perspective

Take a minute and do the following exercise:

Imagine yourself walking on a dock next to a huge ship, any ship, a cruise ship, a war ship, or cargo ship. The ship represents your problem, whether it is one of health, finances, or family, and it is set to sail across the Atlantic Ocean.

In the space below write down what this ship represents to you:

_____

_____

_____

_____

_____

Write out what you can see now that you are on the ship. What are the possibilities you see now that your perspective has changed?

Ex: I can now see areas in my life that I can easily make changes that won't disrupt my lifestyle—like drinking a glass of water as soon as I get up in the morning.

_____

_____

_____

_____

_____

_____

Scenario #1: Ate something I feel bad about:

- Don't worry!

- Identify the situation, then Rewind, Review, and Reevaluate.

- Eat according to your guidelines at the next meal. Remember nothing is a total loss.

Scenario #2: Overeating on vacation/during holiday seasons:

- Don't worry!

- Take the next week and eat according to your guidelines. Reset your focus on eating lean proteins and non-starchy vegetables. Give your body at least a week to readjust.

- Practice Rewind, Review, and Reevaluate.

- Prepare for the next trip or holiday by making a plan.

Scenario #3: Regaining all or most of your weight back:

- Time to worry.

- Make a plan that includes what worked before. Remember, you have been a good loser, and a good re-gainer. Just because you regained your weight does not mean a diet focusing on protein and produce did not work. Separate what worked and how you sabotaged yourself.

- Practice Rewind, Review, and Reevaluate.

- Get support, get help. ASAP!

- Begin anew by establishing some small changes.

Plan your course correction

Which Scenario	Identigy the Situation	Course Correction
Vacation #2	Went on a cruise and overate and drank	This week, eating protein and produce and going to the gym.

Small Changes, Big Results

The key is to make a choice or a change that is important to you and for you to be intentional about your change. The change has to be easy, minimal, and attainable. A small change can be as simple as adding 30 seconds on to your five-minute walk every day. It can be a simple food swap, replacing a soda with water.

Sometimes the thought of making a whole lifestyle change is overwhelming.

Have you ever been on the dock next to a big ship? The sight of the ship is more than the eye can take in all at once. Change can feel this way. After we've tapped into our personal power, it's time to get on that ship! We don't have to make all the changes now. We can take them one step at a time.

Step 1: Make a list of the behaviors you can change today that would take little or no effort.

- Add in 5 extra minutes of walking a day   Take the stairs after lunch (two flights)

- Drink more water   Fill a 16oz water bottle and finish it at lunch

_____

_____

_____

Step 2: Once you've implemented a small change, take some time and evaluate how it's going. Answer the following questions:

1.   Did the change take more time than I thought it would?

2.   What did I like about making that change?

3.   What would I change about the choice I made?

4.   Is there room for me to make additional changes?

5.   How am I feeling about the changes? Good? Empowered?

Rewind, Return, and Reevaluate

It's not enough just to course correct. If we want to go beyond the diet and finally change our relationship to food, we have to learn something about ourselves and our behavior. When we do that we can use what we learned for the next time.

Powerful Process: Rewind, Return, and Reevaluate

Monday Morning Quarterback

Rewind: In your mind, rewind the event or events. Let yourself go back to the moment, the occasion or situation.

Return: As you think of the event, return to it by visualizing yourself there. Ask yourself some questions:

What was I thinking?

What was I feeling?

Was I under stress?

Reevaluate: While you are thinking, look at the scene before you and ask the following questions:

Was there anything I could have done differently?

What did I do that was constructive?

What did I do that was destructive?

Step 2: Create a plan for the next time you are in the same or a similar situation.

_____

_____

_____

_____

_____

Section Two: Aligning

Aligning Personal Power
Aligning Your Self-Image
Aligning Your Motivation

SECTION TWO IS DEVOTED TO the alignment of self. In the past, when you've started down the road of a diet program or a wellness program, it was all about getting to the destination. It was about the number on the scale or improving your health in some way. When we take the time to think about who we are and what motivates us toward achievement, we align or position ourselves for success. In these chapters, you will tap into your personal power and create a positive self-image and learn to use intrinsic motivation to power your success.

Chapter Five:
Aligning Personal Power

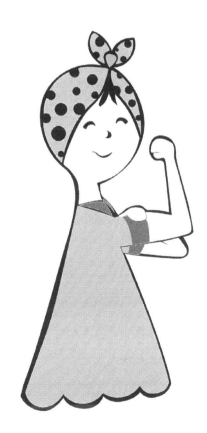

Powerful Process: Tapping into Personal Power

Here is an exercise designed to have you tap into your personal power.

Step 1

Remember a time you felt powerful, confident, loved, and in control. Basically, a time you felt the way you want to feel all the time especially around food. Write about that time in the space below. Be sure to describe how you felt.

Example: I remember when I graduated from college. My goal was to have a job immediately upon graduation. I felt confident, powerful, and successful because I achieved the goal I set out for myself.

_____

_____

_____

Step 2

Now let's put an image to what you felt at that time. The mind works well with images.

Example: The image I associate with feeling confident, powerful, and successful is an eagle. It represents something that is powerful and confident. When I watch an eagle fly, I get the sense of freedom. What is your image? List the first one that comes to mind.

_____

_____

_____

Step 3

Activate your image; take a breath and breathe in while thinking of your image; count to 6 and then exhale. Repeat this, thinking of your image and the feeling you felt in Step 1.

For example: Breathe in thinking of eagle and exhale saying, "confident, powerful, and free."

Step 4

Now that you have your image, take a moment and write down a few ideas of how you can remind yourself of your image. For example: Create a screen saver with your image. Use it at work to remind yourself of your personal power.

_____

_____

_____

Step 5:

Think about times in the past or situations you may be planning in the future. Image using your image to tap into your personal power. For example, if you are planning a trip back home, and in the past, you've found yourself falling back into your childhood habits or roles. How might tapping into your personal power change the outcome? Use the space below and come up with a game plan on how you might tap into your personal power to help you in the situation.

_____

_____

_____

Chapter Six:
Aligning Self Image

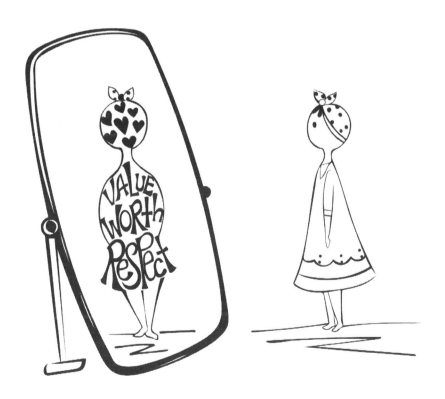

"I am loving, caring, and compassionate."

Powerful Process: Self Image

Step 1: What is your opinion of yourself? Who do you say you are? Who do you feel you are? In the space below write down how you've been talking about yourself. Maybe your friends and family have pointed out self-deprecating things you say about yourself.

    For example, *I am a wife, mother, daughter, friend, and tax accountant. I can't get organized enough to plan my meals, and when it comes to dieting, I am a failure. I could never do that, I am not the smartest tack in the box.*

Step 2: Take a moment and rephrase your statements. Use S.W.A.T. to ask yourself some questions about your self-image. Stop What you are doing, Ask yourself some questions, and Take action.

Self-Talk	S.W.A.T. Question	Rephrase
Ex: I can't get organized	What gets in my way?	At times I find it difficult to organize my food, especially when I have demands at work.

Step 3: Now change your paradigm by changing your focus. Make a list of your positive attributes in one column. In the second column, make a list of how you can use that attribute in other situations that involve making healthy choices.

My Strengths	How to transfer my strength to positive health behaviors
Ex: I am organized when it comes to work. I am a loyal friend; people can count on me. I am bold when it comes to adventure	I have available foods that fit within my guidelines. I am faithful to myself by acknowledging when I am using food as a distraction. I am able to say "no" and be okay with the feelings I may be experiencing.

Step 4: Once you are done, write down five to ten reasons why you are important and why are your goals are important.

1.	
2.	
3.	
4.	
5.	
6.	
7.	
8.	
9.	
10.	

Imagine Who You Are

Take a moment and consider thinking about your self-image: how you view yourself and your abilities. Visualize yourself being successful, doing the things you want, whether it's wearing a certain size of clothing or running a race or getting that job promotion. When we consider something, even before we take action, we open ourselves up to possibilities we never imagined.

Chapter Seven: Motivation

1. Identify the "reason" weight loss is important
2. Focus on what you want rather than don't want
3. Triggers for past weight gain
4. Changing from extrinsic motivation to intrinsic
5. Tapping into intrinsic motivation

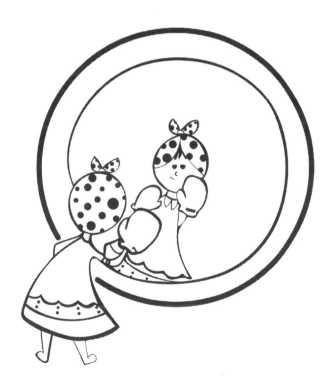

Stop beating yourself up—Focus on what's important about the journey

Three Reasons for wanting to lose weight

Take a minute and write down three reasons you want to lose weight.

List three reasons for wanting to lose weight:
1. _____
2. _____
3. _____

Are these three reasons intrinsic or extrinsic?

Powerful Process: Focus on what you want

Often it is easier to identify what you don't want. We focus our attention on the things we are afraid will happen or the things we hope don't happen. For example, "I don't want to regain my weight," "I don't want to feel hungry," "I don't want to have to watch my diet." Take a minute and list all the things you don't want; then in the other column list what you do want.

What I Don't Want or Can't Have	What I do want
Ex: I don't want to ruin what I've already accomplished. I don't want to cheat on my diet	I want to continue being aware of my goals and making choices that are constructive. I want to choose healthy foods like protein and produce.

Contemplative exercise: Sit quietly and picture yourself at your goal weight, engaging in the activities that bring you joy. See yourself making constructive choices and feeling powerful, free, and happy. Using the image you created for personal power, breath in that image and all that it stands for. Focus all the while on what you want, how you want to show up for yourself every day and in every situation.

Triggers for past weight gain:

Take some time before moving on to identify these factors. Ask yourself, "Were the reasons I regained weight fact or feeling?" "What will I do differently this time?"

What were the reasons I stopped my diet/got derailed in the past?	How will I overcome those reasons this time?	How am I different this time? How are the circumstances different this time?

Take a minute and write out your motivational drivers for wanting to lose weight.

Powerful Process: Moving Toward Intrinsic Motivation

Step 1: Cultivate a positive mind.

What do I want?

_____

Step 2: In order to foster intrinsic motivation, reflect on the benefits of the behavior change or weight loss. Answer these questions:

How will losing weight/maintaining my weight improve my life?

_____

What's so important about that?

_____

Step 3 is to identify tangible goals.

Types of Goals	Target Goal	Timeline	What can I do now?
Health Related Goal	Lose 20 pounds	January 25th	Begin eating foods that are in my lane
Physical Goals	Run a 5 K	March 17th	Begin walking for 10 minutes each day
Personal Goals	Go to Spain	June 1st	Save money, plan itinerary.

Powerful Process: Tapping into Intrinsic Motivation

Step 1: Identify which type of motivation is driving you right now.

Why do you want to reduce your weight? What's important to you?

_____

What health goals do you have? Extrinsic

_____

_____

What events or occasions are on the horizon? Extrinsic

_____

_____

Intrinsic Motivation: How something makes you feel. What do you value about that feeling? What is important about that feeling?

_____

_____

_____

Step 2: Making it a priority

Pictures say a million things, and our mind organizes around pictures. Take some time and cut out pictures from a magazine or an online source that represent how you want to be when you are a healthy weight. For example, I want to hike, feel confident, and choose healthy foods. The pictures I might have are a person hiking, someone looking confident, maybe on top of a hill, and pictures of protein and produce. Put your pictures on a vision board. Once it is finished, put it in a place that you see every day. The bathroom mirror is best because you spend the most amount of time there.

Use the blank sheet of paper on the next page to create your vision board. These are things you want, how you see yourself, what's important to you. Remember to keep it positive.

Section Three: Refining

Refine your understanding of drivers for behaviors
Refine your awareness of hidden agendas
Refine your thinking

THIS SECTION IS DESIGNED TO give you a deeper understanding of the drivers behind your behaviors. Many people ask, "Why do I do what I do?" This secion is about learning how our reward center influences choices, and willpower is not to blame. Section Three is about fine-tuning, dialing in, and reaching for overall self improvement. The more we understand our drivers, the more we can change and rewrite our scrips and ultimately rewire the brain so you no longer give your power away to food.

Chapter Eight: Physical Drivers

It's Not "Just" that I love food

1. Desire versus Distraction
2. Tolerating Discomfort
3. Changing Habits

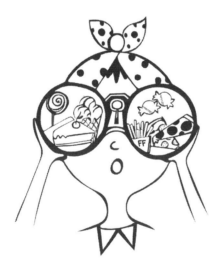

We are constantly looking for opportunities
to improve how we feel

Desire	Distraction
• See Food • Smell Food • Environment/situation • Permission (vacation, birthday) • Reward (I deserve it)	I feel uncomfortable and want to feel better • Sad Happy • Lonely Connected • Tired Energized • Angry Calm • Hurt Loved • Stressed Peace

When you are in a situation where you want something that is outside your guidelines, find out what it is you are experiencing: desire or distraction?

Below identify situations where you felt either desire or distraction.

Situation	Desire	Distraction
Ex: At a wedding and see the wedding cake.	Yumm, it looks so good. I want to try it.	
Ex: Home from work, feeling tired and stressed at my boss and the new deadline.		What will make me feel better? Pizza, cake, French fries. I want to be relaxed, calm, and comforted

Every situation is different, and depending on many factors you may experience a variety of tolerance levels for discomfort. Use the chart below to identify your tolerance level. Each and every one of us can tolerate wanting and not getting. Each and every one of us can tolerate being uncomfortable, experiencing distress without turning to food to distract. Use the chart to monitor your tolerance level. Each time your practice tolerating desire or distraction, you will become stronger and able to tolerate more and more. You might even find that you can tolerable more than you thought.

Desire: What's the situation?	Not tolerable 0-1-2-3-4-5 Tolerable	Distraction: What am I feeling?	Not tolerable 0-1-2-3-4-5 Tolerable

Powerful Process: Breaking Old Habits

Habits are behaviors we do for a reason. Over the years of using food for comfort, relaxation, or joy, we begin to react to situations, and the feelings associated with those situations, using food. Eventually, that coping strategy becomes automatic, and we call the automatic behavior a habit.

A habit cycle has three parts:

1. The cue or trigger: This can be time, place, people, situations and emotions.

2. Routine: This is the behavior, which includes food.

3. Reward: How you feel when you begin to eat the food or engage in the behavior.

What can you do differently and still achieve some reward?

When a habit is established, it is out of a need for a reward. The key is to change the behaviors and keep the reward.

Cue/Trigger	Routine	Reward
Time: 3 P.M. Place: at work People: alone in cubby Situations: Work (wedding, holidays, family reunion, etc.) Emotions: Tired, frustrated, overwhelmed	I get up, walk to the vending machine, get a candy bar, talk to Jim, walk back to my desk, and eat the candy Things to try differently: Go for a walk, take more breaks, get a cup of tea or bring a healthy snack to work. Make a point to talk with co-workers	I feel relaxed Calm Energized

Use the formula below to help you identify possible changes to your behavior.

What can you do differently and still achieve the reward?

When (cue) _____ happens,

I will (behavior) _____ instead.

Chapter Nine: Hidden Agendas

1. Describe yourself as food
2. Describe yourself as a behavior
3. Getting needs met
4. Does my behavior have a purpose?

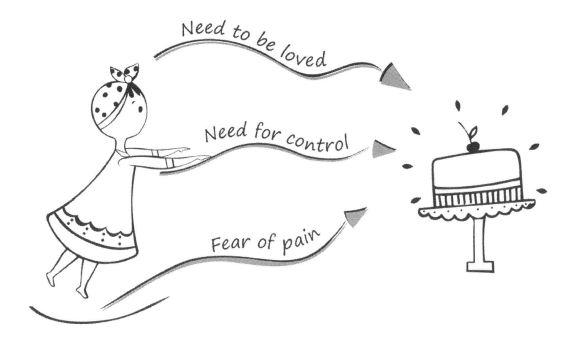

Powerful Process: Hidden Agendas and Needs

Sometimes we have been doing a behavior so long that we forget why we started it in the first place. Hidden agendas are like steps taken to get a need met. Unmet needs ultimately drive our behaviors.

Agenda items include:

- Avoiding physical discomfort

- Avoiding uncomfortable feelings

- Proving you have control and autonomy (over-controlling, worrying)

- Avoiding the risk of getting healthy

- Avoiding feeling deprived

- Avoiding conflict

Needs that may not be getting met include:

- The need for love and belonging

- The need for safety

- Need for autonomy or control

- Need for self-fulfillment and personal growth

Exercise 1:

Describe yourself as any food item you want. Why this food?

Example: I would be cake. Cake is always invited to the party, everyone loves cake.

Food item and why	Agenda	Need	Options for getting that need met
Cake: always included	Avoid uncomfortable feelings of shyness	The need for belonging	Reach out to friends or join a group of people with similar interests.

Exercise 2:

Describe yourself as a behavior.

How do you feel when you do this behavior?

Example: Shopping. When I shop, I have an opportunity to "hang out" with other people, and I feel relaxed.

Behavior: How it feels	Agenda	Need	Options for getting that need met
Shopping: relaxing and social	Avoiding uncomfortable feelings and being alone	Comfort, fulfillment, belonging	Sooth myself by treating myself to a warm bath or herbal tea. Get involved in volunteer work or church organizations.

Does my behavior have a purpose?

All behavior has a purpose. Is our behavior a result of connection or protection? Sometimes we use our weight as a form of protection. Exploring this possibility will help you identify possible reasoning for weight gain and regain.

Take some time and reflect on your life. Answer these questions:

1. When did I begin to gain weight? Or when did I begin to use food as a coping strategy?

2. In the past I have gained and lost weight. What were the triggers for weight regain?

3. Growing up, were there any unusual circumstances in my childhood? Things to consider are disruptive households, divorce, alcoholism, abuse, disappointments, etc.

4. When thinking of your childhood circumstances, remember how you felt during those times? Can you draw a relationship to your behaviors now and your experiences then?

Remind yourself that the past is not happening right now.

5. Finally, write out how you are going to heal the past and move forward with your health and wellbeing. For example, write a letter to your past self, forgiving yourself. Maybe reflect on the hurt you've been holding and decide to write it on a piece of paper and burn it. When we finally decide to let go of negative emotions we create more energy and space in our lives for the things that are most important.

Chapter Ten:
Chatter that Doesn't Matter

1. Identify sound bites

2. Rewrite your story

3. Changing negative thought patterns

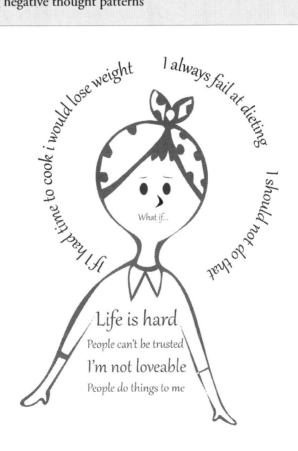

Powerful Process: Identifying Sound Bites

Step 1:

Throughout our lives, we collect messages from people around us: parents, teachers, friends, and bosses. Sometimes we hold onto these messages, and they become the story we tell ourselves. I call these bits of information "sound bites." Just as we have collected negative sound bites, we have also experienced positive sound bites. If your story is a negative one, rewrite it!

In one column write down the negative sound bites you're holding onto, then in the second column think of a sound bite that disputes the negative one.

Collected Sound Bites (Negative)	Ignored Sound Bites (Positive)
I am not liked very well. No one ever invites me to parties or to the movies. I can never stick to a diet. Nothing ever works for me.	Once a month, my friends and I get together for dinner. When I call my friends, they seem to enjoy getting together with me. I have been on many diets and have lost weight. I've been able to maintain my lower weight for short periods of time

Step 2:

In the space below, write your new story based on positive sound bites you used to ignore.

Powerful Process: Chatter that Doesn't Matter

We all engage in automatic thinking to some degree. The question is how much of our thinking can we manage, control, or change? All of it! Below is an outline of thinking patterns, emotions, and beliefs Read through them and identify your most consistent pattern. Then when you find yourself engaging in these patterns, reconstruct that thinking.

4 Ps	Thought	Emotion	Belief
Perception of Danger	• What if • Catastrophic • Jumping to conclusions	• Scared • Fear • Nervous • Anxious	Endangerment: Threatened, intimidated Life is hard; people lie or are out to get you.
Perfectionism	• All or nothing • Comparisons • Should's • Personally	• Mad • Jealously • Inferiority • Frustration • Worthlessness	Rejection: disapproval, judgment, feel criticized I'm not loved. People judge me. I am not capable.
Pessimism	• Overgeneralizations • Dwell on the past • Maximize the negatives	• Hopeless • Depressed • Sad	Neglect: Emotional or physical needs not being met. My feelings don't matter. I'm not important.
Placing Blame	• Minimize your role • Blame circumstances • Need to be right • Need for fairness	• Helpless • Victim • Anger	Betrayal: deceived or manipulated I can't trust others. Life isn't fair. I am not to blame/not my fault.

Powerful Process: Changing Thoughts

We all engage in automatic thinking to some degree. The question is how much of our thinking can we manage, control, or change? Take some time each day and identify your thought patterns and emotions. Spend some time focusing on the underlying belief that may be driving your thinking. Using the chart below, begin to change and restructure a thought to something more positive.

Situation or Trigger	Thought Pattern	Emotion	Belief	Change
I am out with friends, and they order pizza and beer. They don't have to watch what they eat. Why do I?	I should be able to do what they do. It's not fair.	Jealousy/Mad Helpless Victim	Rejection: I'm not capable. I'm judged. Betrayal: Life isn't fair.	I know what is good for my body and what isn't. I am capable of making the right decisions for myself.

Congratulations for finishing this workbook! The journey of changing your relationship to food is a journey in self-discovery. You may have experiences some ups and downs along the way. That is normal. If you found that you needed help or guidance, please know our online community is the place to ask questions, get ideas, and receive support. Need something more personal? Just email me directly.

smaceyphd@gmail.com

Susan@gobeyondthediet.com

www.keepingweightoffforever.com or www.susanmaceyphd.com

Facebook: @Susan Macey PhD

Facebook group: @ Go Beyond the Diet group

Made in the USA
San Bernardino, CA
06 November 2018